COMPREHENSIVE GUIDE ON CANCER OF THE LUNGS: Essential guide on prevention, treatment and management of lung cancer and other respiratory tract disease.

Jose C. Ellison

Table of content.

Chapter 1

General Concept.

1.Upper Respiratory Diseases: Normal Cold, Sinusitis, Pharyngitis, Epiglottitis and Laryngotracheitis

Reasons for upper respiratory tract disease

Most upper respiratory diseases are of viral etiology. Epiglottitis and laryngotracheitis are exemptions with extreme cases probably brought about by Haemophilus influenzae type b. Bacterial pharyngitis is frequently brought about by Streptococcus pyogenes

Normal Specialists of Respiratory Diseases.

Pathogenesis: Organic entities gain passage to the respiratory parcel by inward breath of drops and attack the mucosa. Epithelial obliteration might follow, alongside redness, edema, discharge and at times an exudate.

Side effects : Beginning side effects of a virus are runny, stodgy nose and wheezing, generally without fever. Other upper respiratory diseases might have fever. Youngsters with epiglottitis might experience issues in breathing, muted discourse, slobbering and stridor. Kids with serious laryngotracheitis (croup) may likewise have tachypnea, stridor and cyanosis.

Microbiologic Analysis: Normal colds can for the most part be perceived clinically. Bacterial and viral societies of throat swab examples are utilized for pharyngitis, epiglottitis and laryngotracheitis. Blood societies are additionally acquired in instances of epiglottitis.

Counteraction and Treatment: Viral contaminations are dealt with apparently. Streptococcal pharyngitis and epiglottitis brought about by H influenzae are treated with antibacterials. Haemophilus influenzae type b antibody is monetarily accessible and is presently an essential part of experience growing up vaccination program.

2. Lower Respiratory tract diseases:
Bronchitis, Bronchiolitis and Pneumonia

Reasons for lower respiratory tract diseases

Causative specialists of lower respiratory contaminations are viral or bacterial. Infections cause most instances of bronchitis and bronchiolitis. In people group obtained pneumonias, the most widely recognized bacterial specialist is Streptococcus pneumoniae. Abnormal pneumonias are cause by such specialists as Mycoplasma pneumoniae, Chlamydia spp, Legionella, Coxiella burnetti and infections. Nosocomial pneumonias and pneumonias in immunosuppressed patients have changeable etiology with gram-negative creatures and staphylococci as dominating living beings.

Pathogenesis: Living beings enter the distal aviation route by inward breath, yearning or by hematogenous cultivating. The microbe duplicates in or on the epithelium, causing irritation, expanded bodily fluid emission, and impeded mucociliary capability; other lung capabilities may likewise be impacted. In serious bronchiolitis, aggravation and rot of the epithelium might hinder little aviation routes prompting aviation route hindrance.

Side effects incorporate hack, fever, chest torment, tachypnea and sputum creation. Patients with pneumonia may likewise display non-respiratory side effects like disarray, migraine, myalgia, stomach torment, sickness, regurgitating and loose bowels.

Microbiologic Analysis: Sputum examples are refined for microorganisms, parasites and infections. Culture of nasal washings is typically adequate in newborn children with bronchiolitis. Fluorescent smudging method can be utilized for legionellosis. Blood societies as well as serologic strategies are utilized for infections, rickettsiae, growths and numerous microorganisms. Catalyst connected immunoassay strategies can be utilized for recognitions of microbial antigens as well as antibodies. Location of nucleotide sections explicit for the microbial antigen being referred to by DNA test or polymerase chain response can offer a fast finding.

Avoidance and Treatment: Suggestive treatment is utilized for most popular contaminations. Bacterial pneumonias are treated with antibacterials. A polysaccharide immunization against 23 serotypes of Streptococcus pneumoniae is suggested for people at high gamble.

Upper Respiratory Infections

Contaminations of the respiratory plot are assembled by their symptomatology and anatomic inclusion. Intense upper respiratory contaminations (URI) incorporate the normal cold, pharyngitis, epiglottitis, and laryngotracheitis. These contaminations are generally harmless, short lived and self-restricted, altho ugh epiglottitis and laryngotracheitis can be serious sicknesses in kids and youthful newborn children. Etiologic specialists related with URI incorporate infections, microbes, mycoplasma and organisms. Respiratory contaminations are more normal in the fall and winter when school begins and indoor swarming works with transmission.

Common cold

Normal colds are the most common substance of every respiratory contamination and are the main source of patient visits to the doctor, as well as work and school non-attendance. Most colds are brought about by infections. Rhinoviruses with more than 100 serotypes are the most well-known microorganisms, causing somewhere around 25% of colds in grown-ups. Covids might be liable for over 10% of cases. Parainfluenza infections, respiratory syncytial infection, adenoviruses and flu infections have all been connected to the normal cold disorder. These organic entities show occasional varieties in frequency. The reason for 30% to 40% of cold disorders has not entirely set in stone.

Pathogenesis

The infections seem to act through direct intrusion of epithelial cells of the respiratory mucosa, yet whether there is genuine obliteration and sloughing of these cells or loss of ciliary movement relies upon the particular living being involved. There is an expansion in both leukocyte penetration and nasal emissions, including a lot of protein and immunoglobulin, recommending that cytokines and resistant components might be liable for a portion of the signs of the normal virus.

Side effects

After a hatching time of 48-72 hours, exemplary side effects of nasal release and block, sniffling, sore throat and hack happen in the two grown-ups and kids. Myalgia and cerebral pain may likewise be available. Fever is interesting. The term of side effects and of viral shedding shifts with the microorganism and the age of the patient. Intricacies are typically uncommon, yet sinusitis and otitis media might follow.

Microbiologic Analysis

The conclusion of a typical virus is normally founded on the side effects (absence of fever joined with side effects of confinement to the nasopharynx). Not at all like hypersensitive rhinitis, eosinophils are missing in nasal emissions. Despite the fact that it is feasible to detach the infections for authoritative finding, that is seldom justified.

Prevention and Treatment

Treatment of the simple normal virus is by and large suggestive. Decongestants, antipyretics, liquids and bed rest normally do the trick. Limitation of exercises to try not to contaminate others, alongside great hand washing, are the best measures to forestall spread of the illness. No immunization is economically accessible for cold prophylaxis.

Sinusitis

Sinusitis is an intense provocative state of at least one of the paranasal sinuses. Contamination assumes a significant part in this difficulty. Sinusitis frequently results from diseases of different locales of the respiratory parcel since the paranasal sinuses are adjoining to, and speak with, the upper respiratory lot.

Causes:

Intense sinusitis most frequently follows a typical cold which is normally of viral etiology. Vasomotor and unfavorably susceptible rhinitis may likewise be predecessor to the advancement of sinusitis. Block of the sinusal ostia because of deviation of the nasal septum, presence of unfamiliar bodies, polyps or growths can incline toward sinusitis. Contamination of the maxillary sinuses may follow dental extractions or an augmentation of disease from the underlying foundations of the upper teeth.

The most well-known bacterial specialists answerable for intense sinusitis are Streptococcus pneumoniae, Haemophilus influenzae, and Moraxella catarrhalis. Different creatures including

Staphylococcus aureus, Streptococcus pyogenes, gram-negative organic entities and anaerobes have additionally been recuperated. Constant sinusitis is regularly a blended contamination of high-impact and anaerobic creatures.

Pathogenesis

Contaminations brought about by infections or microorganisms weaken the ciliary action of the epithelial covering of the sinuses and expanded mucous discharges. This prompts impediment of the paranasal sinusal ostia which hinders seepage. With bacterial duplication in the sinus cavities, the bodily fluid is switched over completely to mucopurulent exudates. The discharge further disturbs the mucosal covering causing more edema, epithelial obliteration and ostial deterrent. At the point when intense sinusitis isn't settled and becomes persistent, mucosal thickening outcomes and the advancement of mucoceles and polyps might result.

Side effects

The maxillary and ethmoid sinuses are most ordinarily associated with sinusitis. The front facing sinuses are once in a while involved and the sphenoid sinuses are seldom impacted. Torment, impression of tension and delicacy over the impacted sinus are available. Disquietude and second rate fever may likewise happen. Actual assessment for the most part isn't exceptional without any than an edematous and hyperemic nasal mucosa.

In simple ongoing sinusitis, a purulent nasal release is the most consistent finding. There may not be torment nor delicacy over the sinus regions. Thickening of the sinus mucosa and a liquid level are typically found in x-beam films or attractive reverberation imaging.

Microbiologic Analysis

For intense sinusitis, the analysis is produced using clinical discoveries. A bacterial culture of the nasal release can be taken yet isn't extremely useful as the recuperated creatures are for the most part tainted by the inhabitant verdure from the nasal section. In constant sinusitis, a cautious dental assessment, with sinus x-beams might be required. An antral cut to get sinusal examples for bacterial culture is expected to lay out a particular microbiologic conclusion.

Prevention and Treatment

Suggestive treatment with analgesics and wet intensity over the impacted sinus torment and a decongestant to advance sinus waste might do the trick. For antimicrobial treatment, a beta-lactamase safe anti-microbial, for example, amoxicillin-clavulanate or a cephalosporin might be utilized. For ongoing sinusitis, when moderate treatment doesn't prompt a fix, water system of the impacted sinus might be essential. Culture from an antral cut of the maxillary sinus can be performed to distinguish the causative creature for choosing antimicrobial treatment. Explicit preventive techniques are not accessible. Appropriate consideration of irresistible or potentially hypersensitive rhinitis, careful rectification to alleviate or stay away from obstacle of the sinusal ostia are significant. Root abscesses of the upper teeth ought to get legitimate dental consideration to keep away from auxiliary disease of the maxillary sinuses.

Pharyngitis

Pharyngitis is an aggravation of the pharynx including lymphoid tissues of the back pharynx and horizontal pharyngeal groups. The etiology can be bacterial, viral and parasitic diseases as well as noninfectious etiologies like smoking. Most cases are because of viral contaminations and go with a typical cold or flu. Type A coxsackieviruses can cause an extreme ulcerative pharyngitis in youngsters (herpangina), and adenovirus and herpes simplex infection, albeit more uncommon, likewise can cause serious pharyngitis. Pharyngitis is a typical side effect of Epstein-Barr infection and cytomegalovirus diseases.

Bunch A beta-hemolytic streptococcus or Streptococcus pyogenes is the main bacterial specialist related with intense pharyngitis and tonsillitis. Corynebacterium diphtheriae causes intermittent instances of intense pharyngitis, as do blended anaerobic diseases (Vincent's angina), Corynebacterium haemolyticum, Neisseria gonorrhoeae, and Chlamydia trachomatis. Flare-ups of Chlamydia pneumoniae (TWAR specialist) causing pharyngitis or pneumonitis have happened in military volunteers. Mycoplasma pneumoniae and Mycoplasma hominis have been related with intense pharyngitis. Candida albicans, which causes oral candidiasis or thrush, can include the pharynx, prompting irritation and torment.

Pathogenesis

Similarly as with normal chilly, viral microbes in pharyngitis seem to attack the mucosal cells of the nasopharynx and oral cavity, bringing about edema and hyperemia of the mucous layers and tonsils. Microbes join to and, on account of gathering A beta-hemolytic streptococci, attack the mucosa of the upper respiratory lot. Numerous clinical indications of disease give off an impression of being because of the resistant response to results of the bacterial cell. In diphtheria, a powerful bacterial exotoxin causes neighborhood irritation and cell putrefaction.

Side effects

Pharyngitis normally gives a red, sore, or "scratchy" throat. An incendiary exudate or films might cover the tonsils and tonsillar support points. Vesicles or ulcers may likewise be seen on the pharyngeal walls. Contingent upon the microorganism, fever and fundamental indications like discomfort, myalgia, or migraine might be available. Front cervical lymphadenopathy is normal in bacterial pharyngitis and trouble in gulping might be available.

Microbiologic Conclusion

The objective in the conclusion of pharyngitis is to recognize cases that are because of gathering A beta-hemolytic streptococci, as well as the more strange and possibly serious diseases. The different types of pharyngitis can't be recognized on clinical grounds. Routine throat societies for microbes are immunized onto sheep blood and chocolate agar plates. Thayer-Martin medium is utilized if N gonorrhoeae is thought. Viral societies are not regularly acquired for most instances of pharyngitis. Serologic investigations might be utilized to affirm the analysis of pharyngitis due to viral, mycoplasmal or chlamydial microorganisms. Fast demonstrative tests with fluorescent immune response or plastic agglutination to recognize bunch A streptococci from pharyngeal swabs are accessible. Quality test and polymerase chain response can be utilized to distinguish surprising organic entities, for example, M pneumoniae, chlamydia or infections yet these systems are not standard analytic techniques.

Counteraction and Treatment

Suggestive treatment is suggested for viral pharyngitis. The exemption is herpes simplex infection

Chapter 2

Lower Respiratory Infections

Lower respiratory tract infections are any infections in the lungs or below the voice box. These include pneumonia, bronchitis, and tuberculosis. Symptoms of lower respiratoryInfections of the lower respiratory tract include bronchitis, bronchiolitis and pneumonia. These syndromes, especially pneumonia, can be severe or fatal. Although viruses, mycoplasma, rickettsiae and fungi can all cause lower respiratory tract infections, bacteria are the dominant pathogens; accounting for a much higher percentage of lower than of upper respiratory tract infections.

Bronchitis and Bronchiolitis

Bronchitis and bronchiolitis involve inflammation of the bronchial tree. Bronchitis is usually preceded by an upper respiratory tract infection or forms part of a clinical syndrome in diseases such as influenza, rubeola, rubella, pertussis, scarlet fever and typhoid fever. Chronic bronchitis with a persistent cough and sputum production appears to be caused by a combination of environmental factors, such as smoking, and bacterial infection with pathogens such as *H influenzae* and *S pneumoniae*. Bronchiolitis is a viral respiratory disease of infants and is caused primarily by respiratory syncytial virus. Other viruses, including parainfluenza viruses, influenza viruses and adenoviruses (as well as occasionally *M pneumoniae*) are also known to cause bronchiolitis.

Pathogenesis

When the bronchial tree is infected, the mucosa becomes hyperemic and edematous and produces copious bronchial secretions. The damage to the mucosa can range from simple loss of mucociliary function to actual destruction of the respiratory epithelium, depending on the organisms(s) involved. Patients with chronic bronchitis have an increase in the number of mucus-producing cells in their airways, as well as inflammation and loss of bronchial epithelium, Infants with bronchiolitis initially have inflammation and sometimes necrosis of the respiratory epithelium, with eventual sloughing. Bronchial and bronchiolar walls are thickened. Exudate made up of necrotic material and respiratory secretions and the narrowing of the bronchial lumen lead to airway obstruction. Areas of air trapping and atelectasis develop and may eventually contribute to respiratory failure.

Symptoms

Symptoms of an upper respiratory tract infection with a cough is the typical initial presentation in acute bronchitis. Mucopurulent sputum may be present, and moderate temperature elevations occur. Typical findings in chronic bronchitis are an incessant cough and production of large amounts of sputum, particularly in the morning. Development of respiratory infections can lead to acute exacerbations of symptoms with possibly severe respiratory distress.

Coryza and cough usually precede the onset of bronchiolitis. Fever is common. A deepening cough, increased respiratory rate, and restlessness follow. Retractions of the chest wall, nasal flaring, and grunting are prominent findings. Wheezing or an actual lack of breath sounds may be noted. Respiratory failure and death may result.

Microbiologic Diagnosis

Bacteriologic examination and culture of purulent respiratory secretions should always be performed for cases of acute bronchitis not associated with a common cold. Patients with chronic bronchitis should have their sputum cultured for bacteria initially and during exacerbations. Aspirations of nasopharyngeal secretions or swabs are sufficient to obtain specimens for viral culture in infants with bronchiolitis. Serologic tests demonstrating a rise in antibody titer to specific viruses can also be performed. Rapid diagnostic tests for antibody or viral antigens may be performed on nasopharyngeal secretions by using fluorescent-antibody staining, ELISA or DNA probe procedures.

Prevention and Treatment

With only a few exceptions, viral infections are treated with supportive measures. Respiratory syncytial virus infections in infants may be treated with ribavirin. Amantadine and rimantadine are available for chemoprophylaxis or treatment of influenza type A viruses. Selected groups of patients with chronic bronchitis may receive benefit from use of corticosteroids, bronchodilators, or prophylactic antibiotics.

Pneumonia

Pneumonia is an inflammation of the lung parenchyma. Consolidation of the lung tissue may be identified by physical examination and chest x-ray. From an anatomical point of view, lobar pneumonia denotes an alveolar process involving an entire lobe of the lung while bronchopneumonia describes an alveolar process occurring in a distribution that is patchy without filling an entire lobe. Numerous factors, including environmental contaminants and autoimmune diseases, as well as infection, may cause pneumonia. The various infectious agents that cause pneumonia are categorized in many ways for purposes of laboratory testing, epidemiologic study and choice of therapy. Pneumonias occurring in usually healthy persons not confined to an institution are classified as community-acquired pneumonias. Infections arise while a patient is hospitalized or living in an institution such as a nursing home are called hospital-acquired or nosocomial pneumonias. Etiologic pathogens associated with community-acquired and hospital-acquired pneumonias are somewhat different. However, many organisms can cause both types of infections.

Bacterial pneumonias

Streptococcus pneumoniae is the most common agent of community-acquired acute bacterial pneumonia. More than 80 serotypes, as determined by capsular polysaccharides, are known, but 23 serotypes account for over 90% of all pneumococcal pneumonias in the United States. Pneumonias caused by other streptococci are uncommon. *Streptococcus pyogenes* pneumonia is often associated with a hemorrhagic pneumonitis and empyema. Community-acquired pneumonias caused by *Staphylococcus aureus* are also uncommon and usually occur after influenza or from staphylococcal bacteremia. Infections due to *Haemophilus influenzae* (usually nontypable) and *Klebsiella pneumoniae* are more common among patients over 50 years old who have chronic obstructive lung disease or alcoholism.

The most common agents of nosocomial pneumonias are aerobic gram-negative bacilli that rarely cause pneumonia in healthy individuals. *Pseudomonas aeruginosa*, *Escherichia coli*, *Enterobacter*, *Proteus*, and *Klebsiella* species are often identified. Less common agents causing pneumonias include *Francisella tularensis*, the agent of tularemia; *Yersinia pestis*, the agent of plague; and *Neisseria meningitidis*, which usually causes meningitis but can be associated with pneumonia, especially among military recruits. *Xanthomonas pseudomallei* causes melioidosis, a chronic pneumonia in Southeast Asia.

Mycobacterium tuberculosis can cause pneumonia. Although the incidence of tuberculosis is low in industrialized countries, *M tuberculosis* infections still continue to be a significant public health problem in the United States, particularly among immigrants from developing countries, intravenous drug abusers, patients infected with human immunodeficiency virus (HIV), and the institutionalized elderly. Atypical *Mycobacterium* species can cause lung disease indistinguishable from tuberculosis.

Aspiration pneumonias

Aspiration pneumonia from anaerobic organisms usually occurs in patients with periodontal disease or depressed consciousness. The bacteria involved are usually part the oral flora and cultures generally show a mixed bacterial growth. *Actinomyces,* *Bacteroides,* *Peptostreptococcus,* *Veilonella,* *Propionibacterium,* *Eubacterium,* and *Fusobacterium* spp are often isolated.

Atypical pneumonias

Atypical pneumonias are those that are not typical bacterial lobar pneumonias. *Mycoplasma pneumoniae* produces pneumonia most commonly in young people between 5 and 19 years of age. Outbreaks have been reported among military recruits and college students.

Legionella species, including *L pneumophila*, can cause a wide range of clinical manifestations. The 1976 outbreak in Philadelphia was manifested as a typical serious pneumonia in affected individuals, with a mortality of 17%. These organisms can survive in water and cause pneumonia by inhalation from aerosolized tap water, respiratory devices, air conditioners and showers. They also have been reported to cause nosocomial pneumonias.

Chlamydia spp noted to cause pneumonitis are *C trachomatis, C psittaci* and *C pneumoniae. Chlamydia trachomatis* causes pneumonia in neonates and young infants. *C psittaci* is a known cause for occupational pneumonitis in bird handlers such as turkey farmers. *Chlamydia pneumoniae* has been associated with outbreaks of pneumonia in military recruits and on college campuses.

Coxiella burnetii the rickettsia responsible for Q fever, is acquired by inhalation of aerosols from infected animal placentas and feces. Pneumonitis is one of the major manifestations of this systemic infection.

Viral pneumonias are rare in healthy civilian adults. An exception is the viral pneumonia caused by influenza viruses, which can have a high mortality in the elderly and in patients with underlying disease. A serious complication following influenza virus infection is a secondary bacterial pneumonia, particularly staphylococcal pneumonia. Respiratory syncytial virus can cause serious pneumonia among infants as well as outbreaks among institutionalized adults. Adenoviruses may also cause pneumonia, serotypes 1,2,3,7 and 7a have been associated with a severe, fatal pneumonia in infants. Although varicella-zoster virus pneumonitis is rare in children, it is not uncommon in individuals over 19 years old. Morality can be as high as 10% to 30%. Measles pneumonia may occur in adults.

Other pneumonias and immunosuppression

Cytomegalovirus is well known for causing congenital infections in neonates, as well as the mononucleosis-like illness seen in adults. However, among its manifestations in immunocompromised individuals is a severe and often fatal pneumonitis. Herpes simplex virus also causes a pneumonia in this population. Giant-cell pneumonia is a serious complication of measles and has been found in children with immunodeficiency disorders or underlying cancers who receive live attenuated measles vaccine. *Actinomyces* and *Nocardia* spp can cause pneumonitis, particularly in immunocompromised hosts.

Among the fungi, *Cryptococcus neoformans* and *Sporothrix schenckii* are found worldwide, whereas *Blastomyces dermatitidis*, *Coccidioides immitis*, *Histoplasma capsulatum* and *Paracoccidioides brasiliensis* have specific geographic distributions. All can cause pneumonias, which are usually chronic and possible clinically inapparent in normal hosts, but are manifested as more serious diseases in immunocompromised patients. Other fungi, such as *Aspergillus* and *Candida* spp, occasionally are responsible for pneumonias in severely ill or immunosuppressed patients and neonates.

Pneumocystis carinii produces a life-threatening pneumonia among patients immunosuppressed by acquired immune deficiency syndrome (AIDS), hematologic cancers, or medical therapy. It is the most common cause of pneumonia among patients with AIDS when the CD4 cell counts drop below $200/mm^3$.

Pathogenesis and Clinical Manifestations

Infectious agents gain access to the lower respiratory tract by the inhalation of aerosolized material, by aspiration of upper airway flora, or by hematogenous seeding. Pneumonia occurs when lung defense mechanisms are diminished or overwhelmed. The major symptoms or pneumonia are cough, chest pain, fever, shortness of breath and sputum production. Patients are tachycardic. Headache, confusion, abdominal pain, nausea, vomiting and diarrhea may be present, depending on the age of the patient and the organisms involved.

Microbiologic Diagnosis

Etiologic diagnosis of pneumonia on clinical grounds alone is almost impossible. Sputum should be examined for a predominant organism in any patient suspected to have a bacterial pneumonia; blood and pleural fluid (if present) should be cultured. A sputum specimen with fewer than 10 while cells per high-power field under a microscope is considered to be contaminated with oral secretions and is unsatisfactory for diagnosis. Acid-fast stains and cultures are used to identify *Mycobacterium* and *Nocardia* spp. Most fungal pneumonias are diagnosed on the basis of culture of sputum or lung tissue. Viral infection may be diagnosed by demonstration of antigen in secretions or cultures or by an antibody response. Serologic studies can be used to identify viruses, *M pneumoniae, C. burnetii, Chlamydia species, Legionella, Francisella*, and *Yersinia*. A rise in serum cold agglutinins may be associated with *M pneumoniae* infection, but the test is positive in only about 60% of patients with this pathogen.

Rapid diagnostic tests, as described in previous sections, are available to identify respiratory viruses: the fluorescent-antibody test is used for *Legionella*. A sputum quellung test can specify *S pneumoniae* by serotype. Enzyme-linked immunoassay, DNA probe and polymerase chain reaction methods are available for many agents causing respiratory infections.

Some organisms that may colonize the respiratory tract are considered to be pathogens only when they are shown to be invading the parenchyma. Diagnosis of pneumonia due to cytomegalovirus, herpes simplex virus, *Aspergillus* spp. or *Candida* spp require specimens obtained by transbronchial or open-lung biopsy. *Pneumocystis carinii* can be found by silver stain of expectorated sputum. However, if the sputum is negative, deeper specimens from the lower respiratory tract obtained by bronchoscopy or by lung biopsy are needed for confirmatory diagnosis.

Prevention and Treatment

Until the organism causing the infection is identified, decisions on therapy are based upon clinical history, including history of exposure, age, underlying disease and previous therapies, past pneumonias, geographic location, severity of illness, clinical symptoms, and sputum examination. Once a diagnosis is made, therapy is directed at the specific organism responsible.

The pneumococcal vaccine should be given to patients at high risk for developing pneumococcal infections, including asplenic patients, the elderly and any patients immunocompromised through disease or medical therapy. Yearly influenza vaccinations should also be provided for these particular groups. An enteric-coated vaccine prepared from certain serotypes of adenoviruses is available, but is only used in military recruits

.   In   AIDS   patients, trimethoprim/sulfamethoxazole, aerosolized pentamidine or other antimicrobials can be given for prophylaxis of *Pneumocystis carinii* infections.

Causes and risk factors for developing respiratory tract disease

Infections in the lower respiratory tract are primarily the result of:

- viruses, as with the flu or respiratory syncytial virus (RSV)
- bacteria, such as *Streptococcus* or *Staphylococcus aureus*
- fungal infections
- mycoplasma, which are neither viruses or bacteria but are small organisms with characteristics of both

In some cases, substances from the environment can irritate or cause inflammation in the airways or lungs, which can lead to an infection. These include:

- tobacco smoke
- dust
- chemicals
- vapors and fumes
- allergens
- air pollution

Risk factors that make a person more likely to develop a lower respiratory tract infection include:

- a recent cold or flu
- a weakened immune system
- being more than 65 years old
- being under 5 years old

- recent surgery

Chapter 3

Lung cancer

Disease is a sickness wherein cells in the body outgrow control. At the point when malignant growth begins in the lungs, it is called cellular breakdown in the lungs. Your lungs are 2 wipe like organs in your chest that are isolated into segments called curves. Your right lung has 3 curves. Your left lung has 2 curves. The left lung is more modest on the grounds that the heart occupies more space on that side of the body.When you breathe in (take in), air enters through your mouth or nose and goes into your lungs through the windpipe (windpipe). The windpipe partitions into tubes called bronchi, which enter the lungs and separation into more modest bronchi. These gap to shape more modest branches called bronchioles. Toward the finish of the bronchioles are little air sacs known as alveoli.

The alveoli ingest oxygen into your blood from the breathed in air and eliminate carbon dioxide from the blood when you breathe out (inhale out). Taking in oxygen and disposing of carbon dioxide are your lungs' primary capabilities.

Cellular breakdown in the lungs is perhaps of the most well-known disease in the US. Skin malignant growth is the most widely recognized type of disease analyzed in the US, trailed by bosom disease (among ladies) and prostate disease (among men). More individuals in the US bite the dust from cellular breakdown in the lungs than some other kind of malignant growth. This is valid for all kinds of people. In the wake of expanding for quite a long time, cellular breakdown in the lungs rates are diminishing broadly, as less individuals smoke cigarettes and as cellular breakdown in the lungs medicines get to the next level. Individuals with cellular breakdown in the lungs are living longer after their conclusion since additional cases are seen as ahead of schedule, when therapy works best.

Cigarette smoking is the main source of cellular breakdown in the lungs. Cellular breakdown in the lungs likewise can be brought about by utilizing different sorts of tobacco (like lines or stogies), breathing handed-down cigarette smoke, being presented to substances like asbestos or radon at home or work, having specific quality transformations (surprising changes made when your body's cells are separating), or having a family background of cellular breakdown in the lungs. Cellular breakdown in the lungs can occur in individuals who never smoked or smoked less than 100 cigarettes in their lifetime.Lung malignant growth is a kind of disease that starts in the lungs. Your lungs are two elastic organs in your chest that take in oxygen when you breathe in and discharge carbon dioxide when you breathe out.

Cellular breakdown in the lungs is the main source of malignant growth passings around the world.

Individuals who smoke have the most serious gamble of cellular breakdown in the lungs, however cellular breakdown in the lungs can likewise happen in individuals who have never smoked. The gamble of cellular breakdown in the lungs increments with the time allotment and number of cigarettes you've smoked. Assuming that you quit smoking, even in the wake of smoking for a long time, you can essentially diminish your possibilities creating cellular breakdown in the lungs.

Symptoms and Causes

What are the symptoms of lung cancer?

Most lung cancer symptoms look similar to other, less serious illnesses. Many people don't have symptoms until the disease is advanced, but some people have symptoms in the early stages. For those who do experience symptoms, it may only be one or a few of these:

- A cough that doesn't go away or gets worse over time.
- Trouble breathing or shortness of breath (dyspnea).
- Chest pain or discomfort.
- Wheezing.
- **<u>Coughing up blood (hemoptysis).</u>**
- **<u>Hoarseness.</u>**
- Loss of appetite.
- Unexplained weight loss.
- Unexplained fatigue (tiredness).
- Shoulder pain.
- Swelling in the face, neck, arms or upper chest (superior vena cava syndrome).
- Small pupil and drooping eyelid in one eye with little or no sweating on that side of your face (Horner's syndrome).

When to see a doctor

Make an appointment with your doctor if you have any persistent signs or symptoms that worry you.

If you smoke and have been unable to quit, make an appointment with your doctor.

Your doctor can recommend strategies for quitting smoking, such as counseling, medications and nicotine replacement products.

Causes

Smoking causes the majority of lung cancers — both in smokers and in people exposed to secondhand smoke. But lung cancer also occurs in people who never smoked and in those who never had prolonged exposure to secondhand smoke. In these cases, there may be no clear cause of lung cancer.

How smoking causes lung cancer

Doctors believe smoking causes lung cancer by damaging the cells that line the lungs. When you inhale cigarette smoke, which is full of cancer-causing substances (carcinogens), changes in the lung tissue begin almost immediately.

At first your body may be able to repair this damage. But with each repeated exposure, normal cells that line your lungs are increasingly damaged. Over time, the damage causes cells to act abnormally and eventually cancer may develop.

Lung cancer is a disease caused by uncontrolled cell division in your lungs. Your cells divide and make more copies of themselves as a part of their normal function. But sometimes, they get changes (mutations) that cause them to keep making more of themselves when they shouldn't. Damaged cells dividing uncontrollably create masses, or tumors, of tissue that eventually keep your organs from working properly.

Lung cancer is the name for cancers that start in your lungs — usually in the airways (bronchi or bronchioles) or small air sacs (alveoli). Cancers that start in other places and move to your lungs are usually named for where they start (your healthcare provider may refer to this as cancer that's metastatic to your lungs).

What are the types of lung cancer?

There are many cancers that affect the lungs, but we usually use the term "lung cancer" for two main kinds: non-small cell lung cancer and small cell lung cancer.

Non-small cell lung cancer (NSCLC)

Non-small cell lung cancer (NSCLC) is the most common type of lung cancer. It accounts for over 80% of lung cancer cases. Common types include adenocarcinoma and squamous cell carcinoma. Adenosquamous carcinoma and sarcomatoid carcinoma are two less common types of NSCLC.

Small cell lung cancer (SCLC)

Small cell lung cancer (SCLC) grows more quickly and is harder to treat than NSCLC. It's often found as a relatively small lung tumor that's already spread to other parts of your body. Specific types of SCLC include small cell carcinoma (also called oat cell carcinoma) and combined small cell carcinoma.

Other types of cancer in the lungs

Other types of cancer can start in or around your lungs, including lymphomas (cancer in your lymph nodes), sarcomas (cancer in your bones or soft tissue) and pleural mesothelioma (cancer in the lining of your lungs). These are treated differently and usually aren't referred to as lung cancer.

What are the stages of lung cancer?

Cancer is usually staged based on the size of the initial tumor, how far or deep into the surrounding tissue it goes, and whether it's spread to lymph nodes or other organs. Each type of cancer has its own guidelines for staging.

Lung cancer staging

Each stage has several combinations of size and spread that can fall into that category. For instance, the primary tumor in a Stage III cancer could be smaller than in a Stage II cancer, but other factors put it at a more advanced stage. The general staging for lung cancer is:

- **Stage 0 (in-situ):** Cancer is in the top lining of the lung or bronchus. It hasn't spread to other parts of the lung or outside of the lung.
- **Stage I:** Cancer hasn't spread outside the lung.
- **Stage II:** Cancer is larger than Stage I, has spread to lymph nodes inside the lung, or there's more than one tumor in the same lobe of the lung.
- **Stage III:** Cancer is larger than Stage II, has spread to nearby lymph nodes or structures or there's more than one tumor in a different lobe of the same lung.
- **Stage IV:** Cancer has spread to the other lung, the fluid around the lung, the fluid around the heart or distant organs.

Limited vs. extensive stage

While providers now use stages I through IV for small cell lung cancer, you might also hear it described as limited or extensive stage. This is based on whether the area can be treated with a single radiation field.

- **Limited stage SCLC** is confined to one lung and can sometimes be in the lymph nodes in the middle of the chest or above the collar bone on the same side.
- **Extensive stage SCLC** is widespread throughout one lung or has spread to the other lung, lymph nodes on the opposite side of the lung, or to other parts of the body.

What is metastatic lung cancer?

Metastatic lung cancer is cancer that starts in one lung but spreads to the other lung or to other organs. Metastatic lung cancer is harder to treat than cancer that hasn't spread outside of its original location.

How common is lung cancer?

Lung cancer is the third most common cancer in the U.S. Health systems report over 200,000 new cases of lung cancer each year.

Risk factors

A number of factors may increase your risk of lung cancer. Some risk factors can be controlled, for instance, by quitting smoking. And other factors can't be controlled, such as your family history.

Risk factors for lung cancer include:

- **Smoking.** Your risk of lung cancer increases with the number of cigarettes you smoke each day and the number of years you have smoked. Quitting at any age can significantly lower your risk of developing lung cancer.
- **Exposure to secondhand smoke.** Even if you don't smoke, your risk of lung cancer increases if you're exposed to secondhand smoke.
- **Previous radiation therapy.** If you've undergone radiation therapy to the chest for another type of cancer, you may have an increased risk of developing lung cancer.

- **Exposure to radon gas.** Radon is produced by the natural breakdown of uranium in soil, rock and water that eventually becomes part of the air you breathe. Unsafe levels of radon can accumulate in any building, including homes.
- **Exposure to asbestos and other carcinogens.** Workplace exposure to asbestos and other substances known to cause cancer — such as arsenic, chromium and nickel — can increase your risk of developing lung cancer, especially if you're a smoker.
- **Family history of lung cancer.** People with a parent, sibling or child with lung cancer have an increased risk of the disease.

Complications

Lung cancer can cause complications, such as:

- **Shortness of breath.** People with lung cancer can experience shortness of breath if cancer grows to block the major airways. Lung cancer can also cause fluid to accumulate around the lungs, making it harder for the affected lung to expand fully when you inhale.
- **Coughing up blood.** Lung cancer can cause bleeding in the airway, which can cause you to cough up blood (hemoptysis). Sometimes bleeding can become severe. Treatments are available to control bleeding.
- **Pain.** Advanced lung cancer that spreads to the lining of a lung or to another area of the body, such as a bone, can cause pain. Tell your doctor if you experience pain, as many treatments are available to control pain.
- **Fluid in the chest (pleural effusion).** Lung cancer can cause

fluid to accumulate in the space that surrounds the affected lung in the chest cavity (pleural space). Fluid accumulating in the chest can cause shortness of breath. Treatments are available to drain the fluid from your chest and reduce the risk that pleural effusion will occur again.

- **Cancer that spreads to other parts of the body (metastasis).** Lung cancer often spreads (metastasizes) to other parts of the body, such as the brain and the bones.

  Cancer that spreads can cause pain, nausea, headaches, or other signs and symptoms depending on what organ is affected. Once lung cancer has spread beyond the lungs, it's generally not curable. Treatments are available to decrease signs and symptoms and to help you live longer.

Prevention

There's no sure way to prevent lung cancer, but you can reduce your risk if you:

- **Don't smoke.** If you've never smoked, don't start. Talk to your children about not smoking so that they can understand how to avoid this major risk factor for lung cancer. Begin conversations about the dangers of smoking with your children early so that they know how to react to peer pressure.
- **Stop smoking.** Stop smoking now. Quitting reduces your risk of lung cancer, even if you've smoked for years. Talk to your doctor about strategies and stop-smoking aids that can help you quit. Options include nicotine replacement products, medications and support groups.
- **Avoid secondhand smoke.** If you live or work with a smoker, urge him or her to quit. At the very least, ask him or her to smoke outside. Avoid areas where people smoke, such as bars and

restaurants, and seek out smoke-free options.

- **Test your home for radon.** Have the radon levels in your home checked, especially if you live in an area where radon is known to be a problem. High radon levels can be remedied to make your home safer. For information on radon testing, contact your local department of public health or a local chapter of the American Lung Association.

- **Avoid carcinogens at work.** Take precautions to protect yourself from exposure to toxic chemicals at work. Follow your employer's precautions. For instance, if you're given a face mask for protection, always wear it. Ask your doctor what more you can do to protect yourself at work. Your risk of lung damage from workplace carcinogens increases if you smoke.

- **Eat a diet full of fruits and vegetables.** Choose a healthy diet with a variety of fruits and vegetables. Food sources of vitamins and nutrients are best. Avoid taking large doses of vitamins in pill form, as they may be harmful. For instance, researchers hoping to reduce the risk of lung cancer in heavy smokers gave them beta carotene supplements. Results showed the supplements actually increased the risk of cancer in smokers.

- **Exercise most days of the week.** If you don't exercise regularly, start out slowly. Try to exercise most days of the week.

Chapter 4

How long can you have lung cancer without knowing?

Cancer can grow in your body for a long time — years — before you know it's there. Lung cancer often doesn't cause symptoms in early stages.

Does vaping cause lung cancer?

You can inhale a number of substances when you vape (use a device to inhale a mist of nicotine and flavoring), including some that are known to cause cancer. Vaping is too new to know all of its long-term effects, but experts believe that it has the potential to cause lung damage.

Can you get lung cancer if you don't smoke?

While smoking is the leading risk factor for lung cancer, up to 20% of people diagnosed have never smoked. That's why it's important to talk to your provider about any concerning symptoms.

Diagnosis and Tests

How is lung cancer diagnosed?

Diagnosing lung cancer can be a multi-step process. Your first visit to a healthcare provider will usually involve them listening to your symptoms, asking you about your health history and performing a physical exam (like listening to your heart and lungs). Since lung cancer symptoms are similar to many other, more common illnesses, you provider may start by getting blood tests and a chest X-ray.

If your provider suspects you could have lung cancer, your next steps in diagnosis would usually involve more imaging tests, like a CT scan, and then a biopsy. Other tests include using a PET/CT scan to see if cancer has spread, and tests of cancerous tissue from a biopsy to help determine the best kind of treatment.

Does a chest X-ray show lung cancer?

X-rays aren't as good as CT scans for showing a tumor in your lungs, especially at earlier stages. Tumors might be too small to see on an X-ray or can be blocked from view by other structures in your body (like your ribs). X-rays can't diagnose lung cancer — they can only show your provider if there's something suspicious that they should look into further.

What tests will be done to diagnose lung cancer?

Tests your healthcare provider might order or perform include blood tests, imaging, and biopsies of fluid or tissue.

Blood tests

Blood tests can't diagnose cancer on their own, but can help your provider check how your organs and other parts of your body are working.

Imaging

Chest X-rays and CT scans give your provider images that can show changes in your lungs. PET/CT scans are usually done to evaluate a concerning finding on a CT scan or after a cancer diagnosis to determine whether cancer has spread.

Biopsy

There are a number of procedures your provider can use to look more closely at what's going on inside your chest. During the same procedures, your provider can take samples of tissue or fluid (biopsy), which can be studied under a microscope to look for cancer cells and determine what kind of cancer it is. Samples can also be tested for genetic changes (mutations) that might affect your treatment.

Procedures used to initially diagnose lung cancer or learn more about its spread include:

- **Needle biopsy**. During this procedure, your provider will use a needle to collect samples of fluid or tissue for testing.
- **Bronchoscopy, thoracoscopy or video-assisted thoracic surgery (VATS).** A provider uses these procedures to look at parts of your lungs and take tissue samples.
- **Thoracentesis.** A provider uses this procedure to take a sample of the fluid around your lungs for testing.
- **Endobronchial ultrasound or endoscopic esophageal ultrasound.** A provider uses these

procedures to look at and biopsy lymph nodes.

- **Mediastinoscopy or mediastinotomy.** A provider uses these procedures to look at and take samples from the area between your lungs (mediastinum).

Molecular tests

As part of a biopsy, your provider might have your tissue sample tested for gene changes (mutations) that special drugs can target as part of your treatment plan. Genes that might have changes that can be targeted in NSCLC include:

- *KRAS.*
- *EGFR.*
- *ALK.*
- *ROS1.*
- *BRAF.*

- *RET.*
- *MET.*
- *HER2.*
- *NTRK.*

Management and Treatment

How is lung cancer treated?

Treatments for lung cancer are designed to get rid of cancer in your body or slow down its growth. Treatments can remove cancerous cells, help to destroy them or keep them from multiplying or teach your immune system to fight them. Some therapies are also used to reduce symptoms and relieve pain. Your treatment will depend on the type of lung cancer you have, where it is, how far it's spread and many other factors.

What medications/treatments are used in lung cancer?

Lung cancer treatments include surgery, radiofrequency ablation, radiation therapy, chemotherapy, targeted drug therapy and immunotherapy.

Surgery

NSCLC that hasn't spread and SCLC that's limited to a single tumor can be eligible for surgery. Your surgeon might remove the tumor and a small amount of healthy tissue around it to make sure they don't leave any cancer cells behind. Sometimes they have to remove all or part of your lung (resection) for the best chance that the cancer won't come back.

Radiofrequency ablation

NSCLC tumors near the outer edges of your lungs are sometimes treated with radiofrequency ablation (RFA). RFA uses high-energy radio waves to heat and destroy cancer cells.

Radiation therapy

Radiation uses high energy beams to kill cancer cells. It can be used by itself or to help make surgery more effective. Radiation can also be used as palliative care, to shrink tumors and relieve pain. It's used in both NSCLC and SCLC.

Chemotherapy

Chemotherapy is often a combination of multiple medications designed to stop cancer cells from growing. It can be given before or after surgery or in combination with other types of medication, like immunotherapy. Chemotherapy for lung cancer is usually given through an IV.

Targeted drug therapy

In some people with NSCLC, lung cancer cells have specific changes (mutations) that help the cancer grow. Special drugs target these mutations to try to slow down or destroy cancer cells. Other drugs, called angiogenesis inhibitors, can keep the tumor from creating new blood vessels, which the cancer cells need to grow.

Immunotherapy

Our bodies usually recognize cells that are damaged or harmful and destroy them. Cancer has ways to hide from the immune system to keep from being destroyed. Immunotherapy reveals cancer cells to your immune system so your own body can fight cancer.

Treatments to ease symptoms (palliative care)

Some lung cancer treatments are used to relieve symptoms, like pain and difficulty breathing. These include therapies to reduce or remove tumors that are blocking airways, and procedures to remove fluid from around your lungs and keep it from coming back.

Side effects of the treatment

Side effects of lung cancer treatment depend on the type of treatment. Your provider can tell you what side effects to expect, and what complications to look out for, for your specific treatment.

Chemotherapy

- Nausea, vomiting.
- Diarrhea.
- Hair loss.
- Fatigue.
- Mouth sores.

- Loss of feeling, weakness or tingling (neuropathy).

Immunotherapy

- Fatigue.
- Itchy rash.
- Diarrhea.
- Nausea, vomiting.
- Joint pain.
- Complications (like pneumonitis, colitis, hepatitis and others) can have additional side effects.

Radiation therapy

- Shortness of breath.
- Cough.
- Pain.

- Fatigue.
- Difficulty swallowing.
- Dry, itchy or red skin.
- Nausea, vomiting.

Surgery

- Shortness of breath.
- Chest wall pain.
- Cough.
- Fatigue.

How do I manage symptoms and side effects?

Your provider can prescribe medications to help manage your symptoms or side effects of treatment. A palliative care specialist or a dietitian can help you manage pain or other symptoms and improve your quality of life while you're in treatment.

Lung cancer screening

You can increase your chances of catching cancer in its earliest stages with screening tests. You're eligible for lung cancer screening if you meet all of these requirements:

- You're between the ages of 50 and 80.
- You either currently smoke or have quit smoking within the last 15 years.
- You have a 20 pack-year smoking history (number of packs of cigarettes per day times the number of years you smoked).

Ask your provider about the benefits and risks of yearly screening.

Outlook / Prognosis

What can I expect if I have lung cancer?

What to expect after a lung cancer diagnosis depends on many factors. For some with early stage cancer, your provider will remove the cancer and you'll need follow up screenings for several years. For many others, it's a process that evolves over time. It may mean doing one type of treatment until it stops being effective, then moving on to another type.

Does lung cancer spread quickly?

How fast lung cancer spreads depends on the type. Of the main types, small cell lung cancer tends to spread faster than non-small cell lung cancer. By the time lung cancer is found, it may have already started spreading to lymph nodes or other organs.

Can lung cancer be cured?

Some types of lung cancer can be considered cured if diagnosed before they spread, though experts don't often use the word "cured" to describe cancer. More common terms are "remission" or "no evidence of disease" (NED). If you're in remission or NED for five years or more, you might be considered cured. There's always a small chance that cancer cells could come back.

What is the survival rate of lung cancer?

The survival rate of lung cancer depends greatly on how far cancer has spread when it's diagnosed, how it responds to treatment, your overall health and other factors. For instance, for small tumors that haven't spread to the lymph nodes, the survival rates are 90% for tumors that are smaller than 1 cm, 85% for tumors between 1 and 2 cm, and 80% for tumors between 2 and 3 cm.

The relative five-year survival rate for lung cancer diagnosed at any stage is 22.9%. The five-year relative survival rates by how much cancer has spread is:

- 61.2% (64% for NSCLC, 29% for SCLC) for cancer that's confined to one lung (localized).
- 33.5% (37% for NSCLC, 18% for SCLC) for cancer that's spread to the lymph nodes (regional).
- 7% (26% for NSCLC, 3% for SCLC) for cancer that's spread to other organs (distant).

Remember that these numbers don't take into account the specific details of your diagnosis and treatment. Thanks to improvements in detection and treatment, the rates of lung cancer deaths have been rapidly coming down in recent years.

What do relative survival rates mean?

Your healthcare provider may share five-year survival rates as a way of explaining how your lung cancer may affect your health five years after diagnosis. These numbers compare the survival rate of someone with lung cancer to someone of the same age in the general population.

Chapter 5

Living With lung cancer

How do I take care of myself?

Self-care is an important part of cancer care. Some ways you can take care of yourself while receiving or recovering from treatment include:

- Bringing a friend or family member with you to appointments if you can. They can help you keep track of the information and options your provider gives you.
- Planning in advance for how you'll feel in the days following treatment. This might include asking for extra help, having meals prepared ahead of time or making sure you have a light schedule.
- Asking your provider about getting proper nutrition even if you don't feel well. Drinking plenty of fluids to stay hydrated. Getting exercise if you can and as recommended by your provider.
- Having important phone numbers handy. You may see several providers and it's helpful to know who to contact if issues come up.

- Considering joining a local or online support group. Being around others who've been where you are can help you get perspective and know what to expect.

If you've completed treatments, support and self-care can still play an important part in moving forward. Don't hesitate to reach out for help or guidance. Make sure you follow up with your provider as recommended.

When should I see my healthcare provider?

Check in with your provider if you have any symptoms that concern you. If you smoke or used to smoke, ask your provider about screening for lung cancer.

What questions should I ask my doctor?

- What are my treatment options?

- What's the best way to take care of myself at home?
- What will treatment be like?
- What are my next steps?
- What are the important numbers for questions or emergencies?
- What side effects should I call you about?
- When should I go to the ER?

Recommendations for people with lung carcer

1. Taking proteins such as egg, beans, soya bean goes a long way in increasing the health state of the daily generated cells.
2. Taking vegetables
3. Go for a targeted drug therapy which slows down or destroys cancer cells
4. Surgery to remove the cancer and nearby lymph node
5. Take nut and but butters
6. Take berries
7. Take much of fruits and vegetables
8. Stop smoking

9. Stop taking alcohol and tobacco containing substances.

NOTE:

A lung cancer diagnosis can bring with it a flood of different emotions. Sometimes the volume of new information can be overwhelming. An important thing to remember is that statistics can't tell you how your treatment will go or what decisions are right for your specific situation.

Enlisting the help of trusted loved ones or a support group can help you consider your options and voice your preferences. Cancer treatment is often a process, and taking care of yourself is one of its most important parts.

www.ingramcontent.com/pod-product-compliance
Lightning Source LLC
Chambersburg PA
CBHW070956250726
48663CB00002B/255